# Disclaimer

It's important to note that I am not a medical professional so the information provided should not be taken as medical advice. Before starting any exercise or nutritional program, it is recommended that you consult with a healthcare professional, especially if you have any pre-existing medical conditions or concerns. This is to ensure that you are physically able to engage in the activities that you have planned and to prevent any potential injuries or health complications. Additionally, it's important to start slowly and gradually increase the intensity and duration of your exercise routine to avoid over-exertion and to allow your body time to adjust. Furthermore, be sure to listen to your body, if you feel pain or discomfort, stop the activity and rest. Always make sure to get professional advice and guidance.

# DO THE EASY FITNESS

## Mastering Carb Cycling: A Comprehensive Guide to Optimal Health and Performance

### Do The Easy Fitness Philosophy

Exercise and Nutrition are two of the most powerful tools we have for improving our physical and mental health. Regular physical activity can help to reduce the risk of chronic diseases such as heart disease, diabetes, and obesity. It can also improve our mood, increase our energy levels, and help us to sleep better. However, despite the numerous benefits of exercise, many people struggle to find the motivation to make it a regular part of their lives. This is where Do The Easy Fitness comes in. It's about motivating yourself and others with everyday Lifestyle changes.

One key to staying motivated is to set specific, achievable goals for yourself. For example, you might set a goal to run a 5K race in the next six months, or to lose a certain amount of weight. Having a clear, measurable goal can help you to stay focused and on track. Additionally, it is essential to find an activity that you enjoy and that fits your lifestyle. Whether it be going for a walk, swimming, cycling, or joining a sports team, finding an activity that you enjoy will make it more likely that you will stick with it.

Another important factor in staying motivated is to have a support system. Having a workout partner or joining a fitness class can help to keep you accountable, and also make the exercise more fun. Also, it is important to remind yourself of the benefits of exercise, not only for the present but also for the future. Regular exercise can help to improve your overall quality of life, both now and in the long-term.

Finally, it is essential to remember that there will be setbacks and obstacles along the way. There will be days when you don't feel like exercising, sticking to your nutritional goals, or when you miss a workout. The important thing is not to let these setbacks discourage you. Instead, focus on getting back on track as soon as possible and not to give up on yourself. Remember that a healthy and active lifestyle is a lifelong commitment and it takes time, patience, and perseverance to make it a regular part of your daily routine.

Also, you have to remember that you may not be able to do what someone else does; but instead, you do what you can do and find what motivates you to be a more fit version of yourself than you were before. For example, I have disabilities that affect my legs so running isn't something for me so I walk when I can or if I'm having a painful day where walking isn't going to work then I flex and contract my leg muscles (isometrics) to the best of my abilities. The whole idea of that is to still exercise areas of your body to the best of **YOUR ABILITY** and not to neglect them. The Do The Easy Fitness Philosophy is a culture and mindset of exercising to the best of **YOUR ABILITY** whether it's by conventional or alternative means to make YOU a more fit YOU!

# DO THE EASY FITNESS

## "Mastering Carb Cycling: A Comprehensive Guide to Optimal Health and Performance"

## Table of contents

**Introduction**

1. What is Carb Cycling?

2. History and Evolution

3. Benefits and Goals

4. Who Can Benefit?

**Chapter 1: The Science Behind Carb Cycling**

1. Understanding Carbohydrates

2. The Role of Insulin

3. Metabolic Flexibility

4. Fat Burning vs. Carbohydrate Burning

**Chapter 2: How Carb Cycling Works**

1.  High Carb Days vs. Low Carb Days

2.  Macronutrient Distribution

3.  Timing Your Carbs

4.  Customizing Your Cycle

**Chapter 3: Designing Your Carb Cycling Plan**

1.  Assessing Your Goals

2.  Determining Your Baseline Diet

3.  Structuring Your Cycle

4.  Sample Plans for Different Goals (Weight Loss, Muscle Gain, Maintenance)

**Chapter 4: Meal Planning and Preparation**

1.  Grocery Shopping Tips

2.  Meal Prep Strategies

3.  Recipes for High Carb Days

4. Recipes for Low Carb Days

## Chapter 5: Exercise and Carb Cycling

1. Matching Carbs with Workouts

2. Strength Training and Muscle Gain

3. Cardio and Fat Loss

4. Recovery and Rest Days

## Chapter 6: Monitoring and Adjusting Your Plan

1. Tracking Progress

2. Adjusting Your Cycle

3. Dealing with Plateaus

4. Long-Term Sustainability

## Chapter 7: Common Challenges and Solutions

1. Cravings and Hunger

2. Social Situations and Eating Out

3. Travel and Busy Schedules

4. Mental and Emotional Aspects

# Chapter 8: Success Stories and Testimonials

1. Case Studies

2. Expert Opinions

3. Personal Anecdotes

4. Lessons Learned

# Chapter 9: Frequently Asked Questions

1. Myths and Misconceptions

2. Practical Tips

3. Troubleshooting

4. Final Advice

# Conclusion

1. Recap of Key Points

2. Encouragement and Motivation

3. Next Steps

4. Resources for Further Reading

# Chapter 1: The Science Behind Carb Cycling

Carb cycling is a dietary strategy that alternates between high and low carbohydrate intake to optimize various aspects of health and performance. To understand how carb cycling works, it is essential to delve into the science behind carbohydrates, insulin, metabolic flexibility, and how the body switches between burning fat and carbohydrates for fuel.

## Understanding Carbohydrates

Carbohydrates are one of the three macronutrients essential for human nutrition, alongside proteins and fats. They are found in a wide range of foods, including grains, fruits, vegetables, and dairy products. Carbohydrates are broken down into glucose, which serves as a primary energy source for the body, particularly for the brain and during physical activity.

1. **Types of Carbohydrates**: Carbohydrates can be categorized into simple and complex carbohydrates. Simple carbohydrates, such as sugars found in fruits and sweets, are rapidly absorbed and provide quick energy. Complex carbohydrates, like those in whole grains and legumes, take longer to digest and offer sustained energy.

2. **Glycemic Index**: The glycemic index (GI) is a measure of how quickly a carbohydrate-containing food raises blood glucose levels. Foods with a high GI cause rapid spikes in blood sugar, while low GI foods result in slower, more stable increases.

3. **Carbohydrate Metabolism**: When you consume carbohydrates, they are digested and converted into glucose, which enters the bloodstream. This glucose can be used immediately for energy, stored as glycogen in the liver and muscles, or converted to fat if consumed in excess.

# The Role of Insulin

Insulin is a hormone produced by the pancreas that plays a critical role in carbohydrate metabolism. It facilitates the uptake of glucose into cells, where it can be used for energy or stored as glycogen. Insulin also inhibits the breakdown of fat for energy, making it a key player in regulating blood sugar levels and energy storage.

1. **Insulin Response**: After consuming carbohydrates, blood glucose levels rise, prompting the pancreas to release insulin. This insulin surge helps transport glucose into cells and lowers blood sugar levels. Different types of carbohydrates can elicit varying insulin responses, with simple sugars generally causing more significant spikes.

2. **Insulin Sensitivity**: Insulin sensitivity refers to how effectively the body's cells respond to insulin. High insulin sensitivity means cells readily absorb glucose, while low sensitivity

(insulin resistance) can lead to elevated blood sugar levels and increased fat storage. Carb cycling can help improve insulin sensitivity by alternating periods of high and low carbohydrate intake.

## Metabolic Flexibility

Metabolic flexibility is the body's ability to switch between using carbohydrates and fats as fuel sources. This adaptability is crucial for maintaining energy balance and optimizing physical performance.

1. **Fuel Utilization**: The body uses different fuels depending on various factors, such as the intensity and duration of physical activity, current diet, and metabolic state. During high-intensity exercise, carbohydrates are the preferred fuel source, while low-intensity activities and rest rely more on fat oxidation.

2. **Adapting to Carb Cycling**: By alternating between high and low carb days, carb cycling promotes metabolic

flexibility. On high carb days, the body becomes efficient at using glucose for energy, while low carb days enhance fat oxidation. This dual capability can improve overall energy utilization and support weight management.

## Fat Burning vs. Carbohydrate Burning

The body can derive energy from both carbohydrates and fats, but the efficiency and preference for these fuels vary based on several factors.

1. **Carbohydrate Burning**: Carbohydrates are a quick and easily accessible energy source, especially during high-intensity activities. The body's glycogen stores, primarily found in muscles and the liver, provide readily available glucose for immediate energy needs.

2. **Fat Burning**: Fat is a more energy-dense fuel source, providing more than double the calories per gram

compared to carbohydrates. However, fat oxidation is a slower process and is predominantly utilized during low to moderate-intensity activities and prolonged exercise.

3. **Balancing Act**: Carb cycling aims to strike a balance between these two fuel sources. High carb days replenish glycogen stores and support intense workouts, while low carb days encourage the body to tap into fat reserves for energy. This balance can enhance overall metabolic efficiency and support various fitness goals.

Understanding the science behind carb cycling provides a solid foundation for implementing this dietary strategy effectively. By recognizing how carbohydrates, insulin, and metabolic flexibility interact, you can tailor your carb cycling plan to suit your individual needs and optimize your health and performance.

# Chapter 2: How Carb Cycling Works

Carb cycling is a strategic approach to managing carbohydrate intake to optimize metabolism, performance, and body composition. This chapter will explore the fundamental principles of carb cycling, including high carb days, low carb days, macronutrient distribution, and the timing of carbohydrate consumption. By understanding these components, you can effectively customize your carb cycling plan to meet your specific goals.

## High Carb Days vs. Low Carb Days

Carb cycling typically involves alternating between high carb days and low carb days. The frequency and duration of these cycles can vary depending on individual goals and activity levels.

1. **High Carb Days**:

    - **Purpose**: High carb days are designed to replenish glycogen stores, enhance performance during intense workouts, and support muscle recovery and growth.

- **Carbohydrate Intake**: On high carb days, carbohydrate intake is significantly increased, often comprising 50-60% of total daily calories. This can range from 2-3 grams of carbohydrates per pound of body weight.

- **Benefits**: Increased carbohydrate intake boosts insulin levels, promoting nutrient delivery to muscles and enhancing recovery. It also supports high-intensity training and can improve metabolic rate by preventing the downregulation of thyroid hormones.

2. **Low Carb Days**:

- **Purpose**: Low carb days aim to promote fat burning, improve insulin sensitivity, and give the digestive system a break from high carbohydrate intake.

- **Carbohydrate Intake**: On low carb days, carbohydrate intake is reduced to around 10-20% of total daily calories, typically 0.5-1 gram of carbohydrates per pound of body weight.

- **Benefits**: Reduced carbohydrate intake lowers insulin levels, encouraging the body to utilize fat as a primary fuel source. It can also help stabilize blood sugar levels and reduce cravings for sugary foods.

## Macronutrient Distribution

In addition to cycling carbohydrate intake, it is essential to consider the distribution of other macronutrients—proteins and fats—on both high and low carb days.

1. **Protein**:

   - **Role**: Protein is crucial for muscle repair, growth, and overall health. It should remain relatively consistent on both high and low carb days to support these functions.

- **Intake**: Aim for 0.8-1 gram of protein per pound of body weight per day, regardless of the carb cycle. This ensures adequate amino acids are available for muscle protein synthesis.

2. **Fats**:

- **Role**: Fats provide a steady source of energy, support hormone production, and aid in the absorption of fat-soluble vitamins. On low carb days, fats play a more significant role in energy provision.

- **Intake**: On high carb days, fat intake should be moderate (20-30% of total calories) to avoid excess calorie consumption. On low carb days, fat intake can be increased (40-50% of total calories) to compensate for the reduced carbohydrate intake and provide sustained energy.

## Timing Your Carbs

The timing of carbohydrate consumption is a critical factor in maximizing the benefits of carb cycling. Proper timing ensures that carbs are available when the body needs them most, such as before, during, and after workouts.

1. **Pre-Workout**:

   - **Purpose**: Consuming carbohydrates before exercise provides readily available energy, enhances performance, and reduces muscle breakdown.

   - **Strategy**: Aim to consume 20-40 grams of easily digestible carbohydrates 30-60 minutes before your workout. Examples include fruits, oats, or a sports drink.

2. **Post-Workout**:

- **Purpose**: Post-workout carbohydrates help replenish glycogen stores, accelerate recovery, and support muscle growth.

- **Strategy**: Within 30 minutes of completing your workout, consume 40-60 grams of carbohydrates along with protein. This combination optimizes glycogen replenishment and muscle repair. Good options include a protein shake with fruit, a smoothie, or a balanced meal with lean protein and starchy carbs.

3. **Throughout the Day**:

- **High Carb Days**: Distribute your carbohydrate intake evenly across meals to maintain steady energy levels and support metabolic function.

- **Low Carb Days**: Focus carbohydrate consumption

around your workout window and consume proteins and fats for the rest of the meals to stabilize blood sugar and promote satiety.

## Customizing Your Cycle

The frequency and duration of high and low carb days can be tailored to individual goals, activity levels, and metabolic responses. Here are some common carb cycling patterns:

1. **Daily Cycle**:

    - **Pattern**: Alternate high carb and low carb days throughout the week.

    - **Example**: High carb on Monday, Wednesday, Friday; low carb on Tuesday, Thursday, Saturday; moderate carb on Sunday.

2. **Weekly Cycle**:

- **Pattern**: Designate specific days of the week as high carb or low carb days.

- **Example**: High carb on Monday, Thursday; low carb on Tuesday, Wednesday, Friday, Saturday; moderate carb on Sunday.

3. **Event-Based Cycle**:

   - **Pattern**: Adjust carbohydrate intake based on specific events, such as workouts, competitions, or rest days.

   - **Example**: High carb on workout days; low carb on rest days or light activity days.

4. **Goal-Oriented Cycle**:

   - **Pattern**: Customize the cycle based on specific goals, such as weight loss, muscle gain, or maintenance.

   - **Example**: For weight loss, implement more low carb days;

for muscle gain, increase the number of high carb days.

Understanding how carb cycling works allows you to create a personalized plan that aligns with your health and fitness objectives. By carefully managing carbohydrate intake, you can optimize energy levels, enhance performance, and achieve your desired body composition.

# Chapter 3: Designing Your Carb Cycling Plan

Creating an effective carb cycling plan requires a thorough assessment of your goals, current diet, and lifestyle. This chapter will guide you through the process of designing a personalized carb cycling plan that aligns with your objectives, whether it's weight loss, muscle gain, or maintenance. We will also provide sample plans for different goals to help you get started.

## Assessing Your Goals

The first step in designing your carb cycling plan is to clearly define your goals. Understanding what you want to achieve will help you tailor your plan to meet your specific needs.

1. **Weight Loss**:

    - **Objective**: Reduce body fat while preserving lean muscle mass.

- **Strategy**: Implement more low carb days to promote fat burning and create a calorie deficit.

2. **Muscle Gain**:

   - **Objective**: Increase muscle mass and strength.
   - **Strategy**: Incorporate more high carb days to support intense workouts, muscle recovery, and growth.

3. **Maintenance**:

   - **Objective**: Maintain current weight and body composition.
   - **Strategy**: Balance high and low carb days to sustain energy levels and prevent weight gain or loss.

4. **Performance Enhancement**:

   - **Objective**: Optimize athletic performance and recovery.
   - **Strategy**: Adjust carbohydrate intake around training sessions

and competitions to ensure peak performance.

## Determining Your Baseline Diet

Before implementing carb cycling, it's essential to establish your baseline diet. This involves calculating your daily caloric needs and macronutrient distribution based on your current weight, activity level, and goals.

1. **Calculating Daily Caloric Needs**:

   - **Basal Metabolic Rate (BMR)**: Estimate the number of calories your body needs at rest.

   - **Total Daily Energy Expenditure (TDEE)**: Multiply your BMR by an activity factor (sedentary, lightly active, moderately active, very active) to determine your daily caloric needs.

2. **Macronutrient Distribution**:

- **Protein**: Aim for 0.8-1 gram of protein per pound of body weight.

- **Fats**: Allocate 20-30% of total daily calories to fats on high carb days and 40-50% on low carb days.

- **Carbohydrates**: Adjust the remaining calories to carbohydrates, with higher intake on high carb days and lower intake on low carb days.

## Structuring Your Cycle

With your goals and baseline diet in mind, you can structure your carb cycling plan. This involves determining the frequency and duration of high and low carb days, as well as planning your meals and snacks accordingly.

1. **Frequency and Duration**:

   - Decide how many high carb and low carb days you will have each week based on your goals.

- Consider starting with a simple pattern (e.g., 3 high carb days, 4 low carb days) and adjust as needed based on your progress and how your body responds.

2. **Meal Planning**:

   - **High Carb Days**: Plan meals that are rich in complex carbohydrates, moderate in protein, and low to moderate in fats. Focus on whole grains, starchy vegetables, fruits, and lean proteins.

   - **Low Carb Days**: Plan meals that are high in protein and healthy fats, with low to moderate carbohydrate intake. Emphasize non-starchy vegetables, lean proteins, nuts, seeds, and healthy oils.

3. **Sample Plans**:

   - **Weight Loss Plan**:

- Monday: High carb (leg day workout)
- Tuesday: Low carb (light cardio)
- Wednesday: Low carb (rest day)
- Thursday: High carb (upper body workout)
- Friday: Low carb (rest day)
- Saturday: Low carb (light cardio)
- Sunday: Moderate carb (active rest)

- **Muscle Gain Plan**:

  - Monday: High carb (full-body workout)
  - Tuesday: Moderate carb (active rest)
  - Wednesday: High carb (upper body workout)
  - Thursday: Low carb (rest day)

  - Friday: High carb (leg day workout)
  - Saturday: Moderate carb (active rest)
  - Sunday: Low carb (rest day)

- **Maintenance Plan**:

  - Monday: Moderate carb (strength training)
  - Tuesday: Low carb (light cardio)
  - Wednesday: High carb (intense workout)
  - Thursday: Moderate carb (active rest)
  - Friday: Low carb (rest day)
  - Saturday: High carb (full-body workout)
  - Sunday: Low carb (rest day)

## Customizing Your Plan

While sample plans provide a good starting point, it's important to customize your carb cycling plan to suit your individual needs and preferences.

1. **Adjusting Based on Progress**:

   - Regularly monitor your progress by tracking body weight, measurements, and performance metrics.

   - Make adjustments to your carb cycle, caloric intake, and macronutrient distribution as needed to ensure continuous progress toward your goals.

2. **Listening to Your Body**:

   - Pay attention to how your body responds to different phases of the carb cycle. Adjust the frequency and duration of high and low carb days based on energy levels, workout performance, and overall well-being.

3. **Flexibility and Sustainability**:

- Ensure your carb cycling plan is flexible and sustainable in the long term. Allow for occasional deviations and adjustments to accommodate social events, travel, and lifestyle changes.

Designing an effective carb cycling plan requires a thoughtful approach that takes into account your goals, baseline diet, and personal preferences. By structuring your cycle, planning your meals, and customizing your approach, you can create a plan that optimizes your health, performance, and body composition.

# Chapter 4: Meal Planning and Preparation

Meal planning and preparation are crucial components of a successful carb cycling plan. This chapter will provide practical tips for grocery shopping, meal prep strategies, and a variety of recipes for both high and low carb days. By mastering these skills, you can ensure that your carb cycling plan is convenient, enjoyable, and sustainable.

## Grocery Shopping Tips

Effective meal planning starts with smart grocery shopping. Here are some tips to help you make the most of your trips to the grocery store:

1. **Plan Ahead**:

   - Create a weekly meal plan that outlines your high and low carb days.
   - Make a detailed shopping list based on your meal plan to

ensure you have all the necessary ingredients.

2. **Shop the Perimeter**:

   - Focus on the perimeter of the grocery store, where fresh produce, lean proteins, dairy, and whole grains are typically located.

   - Minimize your time in the aisles with processed and packaged foods.

3. **Choose Whole Foods**:

   - Opt for whole, unprocessed foods that are rich in nutrients and free from added sugars and unhealthy fats.

   - Prioritize fresh fruits and vegetables, lean meats, fish, eggs, nuts, seeds, and whole grains.

4. **Read Labels**:

- Pay attention to food labels to avoid hidden sugars, unhealthy fats, and artificial additives.
- Look for products with minimal ingredients and no added sugars or trans fats.

## Meal Prep Strategies

Meal prep can save time, reduce stress, and ensure you stick to your carb cycling plan. Here are some strategies to help you get started:

1. **Batch Cooking**:

- Prepare large batches of staple foods, such as grilled chicken, roasted vegetables, quinoa, and brown rice, that can be used in various meals throughout the week.
- Store cooked foods in portioned containers for easy access.

## 2. **Portion Control**:

- Use portion control containers or a food scale to measure and divide your meals into appropriate portions based on your daily macronutrient goals.
- Label containers with the day and meal type (e.g., high carb lunch, low carb dinner) to keep your meals organized.

## 3. **Quick and Easy Recipes**:

- Choose recipes that are simple to prepare and require minimal ingredients and cooking time.
- Utilize kitchen tools like slow cookers, pressure cookers, and sheet pans to streamline the cooking process.

## 4. **Variety and Balance**:

- Incorporate a variety of foods and flavors into your meal plan to keep your meals interesting and nutritionally balanced.

- Rotate different protein sources, vegetables, and grains to ensure a diverse intake of nutrients.

**Recipes for High Carb Days**

Here are some delicious and nutritious recipes for high carb days:

1. **Breakfast: Overnight Oats with Berries and Almonds**

   - **Ingredients**:
     - 1 cup rolled oats
     - 1 cup almond milk
     - 1/2 cup mixed berries
     - 1 tablespoon chia seeds
     - 1 tablespoon sliced almonds
     - 1 teaspoon honey (optional)
   - **Instructions**:

- In a jar or container, combine the oats, almond milk, chia seeds, and honey.
- Stir well and refrigerate overnight.
- In the morning, top with mixed berries and sliced almonds before serving.

## 2. **Lunch**: **Quinoa Salad with Chickpeas and Avocado**

- **Ingredients**:
  - 1 cup cooked quinoa
  - 1/2 cup canned chickpeas, rinsed and drained
  - 1/2 avocado, diced
  - 1/2 cup cherry tomatoes, halved
  - 1/4 cup cucumber, diced
  - 2 tablespoons chopped fresh parsley
  - 2 tablespoons lemon juice
  - 1 tablespoon olive oil

- Salt and pepper to taste
- **Instructions**:
  - In a large bowl, combine the cooked quinoa, chickpeas, avocado, cherry tomatoes, cucumber, and parsley.
  - In a small bowl, whisk together the lemon juice, olive oil, salt, and pepper.
  - Pour the dressing over the salad and toss to combine.

3. **Dinner: Grilled Chicken with Sweet Potato and Asparagus**

- **Ingredients**:
  - 2 boneless, skinless chicken breasts
  - 2 medium sweet potatoes, peeled and cubed
  - 1 bunch asparagus, trimmed
  - 2 tablespoons olive oil
  - 1 teaspoon garlic powder
  - 1 teaspoon paprika

- Salt and pepper to taste

- **Instructions**:

  - Preheat the grill to medium-high heat.

  - Toss the sweet potato cubes with 1 tablespoon of olive oil, garlic powder, paprika, salt, and pepper. Spread on a baking sheet and roast in the oven at 400°F (200°C) for 25-30 minutes, or until tender.

  - Drizzle the asparagus with the remaining olive oil and season with salt and pepper.

  - Grill the chicken breasts for 6-7 minutes per side, or until fully cooked. Grill the asparagus for 3-4 minutes, or until tender.

  - Serve the grilled chicken with roasted sweet potatoes and asparagus.

## Recipes for Low Carb Days

Here are some tasty and satisfying recipes for low carb days:

1. **Breakfast: Spinach and Feta Omelette**

    - **Ingredients**:
        - 3 large eggs
        - 1/2 cup fresh spinach, chopped
        - 1/4 cup crumbled feta cheese
        - 1 tablespoon olive oil
        - Salt and pepper to taste
    - **Instructions**:
        - In a bowl, whisk the eggs with salt and pepper.
        - Heat the olive oil in a non-stick skillet over medium heat.
        - Pour the eggs into the skillet and cook for 1-2 minutes, or until the edges begin to set.

- Add the spinach and feta cheese to one half of the omelette.

- Fold the omelette in half and cook for another 1-2 minutes, or until the eggs are fully set and the cheese is melted.

2. **Lunch: Zucchini Noodles with Pesto and Grilled Chicken**

- **Ingredients**:
    - 2 medium zucchinis, spiralized
    - 1/2 pound chicken
    - 1/4 cup pesto sauce
    - 1 tablespoon olive oil
    - Salt and pepper to taste

- **Instructions**:
    - Heat the olive oil in a large skillet over medium heat.
    - Add the chicken and cook for 6-7 minutes per side, or

until there is no pink. Make sure it is fully cooked.

- Season with salt and pepper.
- In the same skillet, add the zucchini noodles and cook for 2-3 minutes, or until slightly tender.
- Toss the zucchini noodles with the pesto sauce and top with grilled chicken before serving.

3. **Dinner: Baked Salmon with Cauliflower Rice and Broccoli**

- **Ingredients**:
  - 2 salmon fillets
  - 1 head of cauliflower, grated into rice-sized pieces
  - 1 head of broccoli, cut into florets
  - 2 tablespoons olive oil
  - 1 teaspoon garlic powder
  - 1 teaspoon paprika

- Salt and pepper to taste

- **Instructions**:

  - Preheat the oven to 400°F (200°C).

  - Place the salmon fillets on a baking sheet and season with salt, pepper, garlic powder, and paprika. Drizzle with 1 tablespoon of olive oil.

  - Arrange the broccoli florets around the salmon and drizzle with the remaining olive oil. Season with salt and pepper.

  - Bake for 15-20 minutes, or until the salmon is cooked through and the broccoli is tender.

  - While the salmon is baking, heat a large skillet over medium heat and add the grated cauliflower. Cook for 5-7 minutes, or until tender.

- Serve the baked salmon with cauliflower rice and roasted broccoli.

Meal planning and preparation are essential for maintaining consistency and success with your carb cycling plan. By following these tips and incorporating a variety of delicious recipes, you can enjoy nutritious and satisfying meals that support your health and fitness goals.

# Chapter 5: Exercise and Carb Cycling

Exercise plays a crucial role in the effectiveness of carb cycling. This chapter will discuss the relationship between exercise and carb cycling, including the types of workouts that complement high and low carb days, how to structure your training program, and tips for maximizing performance and recovery.

## The Relationship Between Exercise and Carb Cycling

Carb cycling and exercise are closely linked, as the strategic intake of carbohydrates can enhance workout performance, support recovery, and improve overall fitness. Here's how carb cycling interacts with different types of exercise:

1. **High-Intensity Workouts**:

   - **Examples**: Weightlifting, sprinting, high-intensity interval training (HIIT)

- **Carb Intake**: High carb days are ideal for high-intensity workouts, as the increased carbohydrate intake provides the necessary energy for intense exercise and supports muscle glycogen replenishment.

2. **Moderate-Intensity Workouts**:

- **Examples**: Steady-state cardio, circuit training, moderate-intensity strength training
- **Carb Intake**: Moderate carb days can be used for moderate-intensity workouts, providing enough carbohydrates to sustain energy levels without overloading.

3. **Low-Intensity Workouts**:

- **Examples**: Yoga, light walking, stretching, active recovery
- **Carb Intake**: Low carb days are suitable for low-intensity workouts, as the body can rely

more on fat stores for energy, promoting fat burning and improving insulin sensitivity.

## Structuring Your Training Program

To optimize the benefits of carb cycling and exercise, it's important to structure your training program to align with your carb cycling schedule. Here's how to create a balanced program:

1. **High Carb Days**:

   - Schedule high-intensity workouts on high carb days to take advantage of the increased energy and glycogen stores.

   - Focus on compound exercises that target multiple muscle groups, such as squats, deadlifts, bench presses, and pull-ups.

2. **Low Carb Days**:

   - Plan low-intensity or rest days on low carb days to allow your body to recover and promote fat burning.

- Incorporate activities like yoga, stretching, or light cardio to maintain mobility and flexibility without depleting energy reserves.

3. **Weekly Training Split**:

- **Example Split for Muscle Gain**:

    - Monday: High carb (full-body workout)
    - Tuesday: Low carb (rest day)
    - Wednesday: High carb (upper body workout)
    - Thursday: Moderate carb (cardio or active recovery)
    - Friday: High carb (lower body workout)
    - Saturday: Low carb (rest day)

- Sunday: Moderate carb (active recovery or light cardio)

- **Example Split for Weight Loss**:

  - Monday: High carb (HIIT workout)
  - Tuesday: Low carb (light cardio)
  - Wednesday: High carb (strength training)
  - Thursday: Low carb (rest day)
  - Friday: High carb (circuit training)
  - Saturday: Low carb (light cardio)
  - Sunday: Moderate carb (active recovery or yoga)

## Tips for Maximizing Performance and Recovery

To get the most out of your carb cycling and exercise program, consider the following tips:

1. **Pre-Workout Nutrition**:

   - Consume a balanced meal or snack that includes carbohydrates and protein 30-60 minutes before your workout.
   - Hydrate adequately to ensure optimal performance and prevent dehydration.

2. **Intra-Workout Nutrition**:

   - For longer or more intense workouts, consider consuming a carbohydrate and electrolyte drink to maintain energy levels and hydration.

3. **Post-Workout Nutrition**:

   - Eat a meal or snack that includes carbohydrates and protein within 30 minutes of completing your workout to replenish glycogen stores and support muscle recovery.

- Aim for a ratio of approximately 3:1 carbohydrate to protein for optimal recovery.

4. **Rest and Recovery**:

- Prioritize sleep and rest days to allow your body to recover and repair.

- Incorporate active recovery activities, such as light walking or stretching, to promote circulation and reduce muscle soreness.

5. **Monitor and Adjust**:

- Track your workouts, energy levels, and progress to identify patterns and make necessary adjustments to your carb cycling and exercise plan.

- Listen to your body and modify your training intensity and

carbohydrate intake based on
how you feel and perform.

Exercise and carb cycling are synergistic components of a comprehensive fitness plan. By understanding the relationship between carbohydrate intake and different types of workouts, structuring your training program effectively, and following tips for performance and recovery, you can achieve your health and fitness goals more efficiently.

# Chapter 6: Monitoring Progress and Adjustments

Tracking your progress and making necessary adjustments are vital for long-term success with carb cycling. This chapter will cover methods for monitoring progress, evaluating the effectiveness of your plan, and making informed adjustments to continue progressing toward your goals.

## Methods for Monitoring Progress

To determine the effectiveness of your carb cycling plan, it's important to use various methods for monitoring progress. Here are some key metrics to track:

1. **Body Weight**:

   - Regularly weigh yourself to monitor changes in body weight. Aim to weigh in at the same time of day, under similar conditions, for consistency.

   - Note that weight can fluctuate due to factors such as water retention, muscle gain, and hormonal changes, so it's important to look at trends over time rather than day-to-day changes.

2. **Body Measurements**:

- Use a tape measure to track changes in body measurements, such as waist, hips, thighs, and arms.

- Measurements can provide a more accurate picture of body composition changes, especially if you're gaining muscle while losing fat.

3. **Progress Photos**:

- Take progress photos at regular intervals (e.g., bi-weekly or monthly) to visually document changes in your body composition.

- Use consistent lighting, angles, and clothing to ensure comparability over time.

4. **Performance Metrics**:

- Track your performance in workouts, including strength, endurance, and overall energy levels.

- Keep a workout log to record exercises, sets, reps, and weights lifted, as well as any notes on how you felt during and after the workout.

5. **Diet and Nutrition**:

- Maintain a food diary or use a nutrition tracking app to log your daily food intake, including macronutrients and calories.

- Review your food logs to ensure you're adhering to your carb cycling plan and making any necessary adjustments.

6. **Health Markers**:

- Monitor health markers such as blood sugar levels, cholesterol, and blood pressure, especially if you have specific health concerns or conditions.
- Regular check-ups with your healthcare provider can help you assess the impact of carb cycling on your overall health.

## Evaluating the Effectiveness of Your Plan

After tracking your progress for several weeks or months, it's important to evaluate the effectiveness of your carb cycling plan. Here's how to assess your progress:

1. **Review Your Goals**:

- Compare your current progress to your initial goals. Have you made significant strides toward achieving them?

- Determine if your goals need to be adjusted based on your current progress and any new insights.

2. **Analyze Trends**:

   - Look for trends in your data, such as consistent weight loss, muscle gain, or performance improvements.

   - Identify any plateaus or setbacks and consider potential reasons for these trends.

3. **Assess Adherence**:

   - Evaluate how well you've adhered to your carb cycling plan, including dietary intake, exercise routine, and lifestyle habits.

   - Identify any areas where adherence may have been challenging and consider strategies to improve consistency.

4. **Feedback from Your Body**:

   - Pay attention to how your body feels and responds to the carb cycling plan. Are you experiencing sustained energy levels, improved performance, and better overall well-being?

   - Consider any negative feedback, such as fatigue, poor recovery, or digestive issues, and explore possible adjustments.

## Making Informed Adjustments

Based on your evaluation, you may need to make adjustments to your carb cycling plan to continue progressing toward your goals. Here are some common adjustments to consider:

1. **Adjusting Carb Cycling Frequency**:

   - If you're not seeing desired results, consider altering the frequency of high and low carb days. For example, you might add an extra high carb day to support muscle gain or reduce the number of high carb days to promote fat loss.

2. **Modifying Macronutrient Ratios**:

- Experiment with different macronutrient ratios to find the optimal balance for your body and goals. This might involve increasing protein intake to support muscle recovery or adjusting fat intake to improve satiety.

3. **Tweaking Caloric Intake**:

- If you're not losing weight as expected, consider reducing your overall caloric intake. Conversely, if you're struggling to gain muscle, you may need to increase your calorie consumption.

4. **Changing Workout Intensity**:

- Adjust the intensity and type of your workouts to better align with your carb cycling plan. For example, increase the intensity of workouts on high carb days or incorporate more low-intensity activities on low carb days.

## 5. **Incorporating Periodic Breaks**:

- Consider taking periodic breaks from strict carb cycling to prevent burnout and promote long-term adherence. This could involve a week of moderate carb intake or a more flexible eating approach during vacations or special occasions.

## Seeking Professional Guidance

If you're unsure about making adjustments or need additional support, consider seeking guidance from a nutritionist, dietitian, or fitness coach. A professional can provide personalized recommendations based on your unique needs, goals, and progress.

Monitoring progress and making informed adjustments are essential components of a successful carb cycling plan. By regularly tracking key metrics, evaluating the effectiveness of your plan, and making necessary adjustments, you can continue to progress toward your health and fitness goals.

# Chapter 7: Overcoming Challenges and Staying Motivated

Carb cycling can present various challenges, from meal planning and adherence to dealing with social situations and maintaining motivation. This chapter will provide practical strategies for overcoming common challenges and staying motivated throughout your carb cycling journey.

## Common Challenges and Solutions

1. **Meal Planning and Preparation**:

   - **Challenge**: Finding time for meal planning and preparation.
   - **Solution**: Set aside a specific day each week for meal prep, batch cooking, and grocery shopping. Use simple recipes and kitchen tools, like slow cookers and meal prep containers, to streamline the process.

2. **Social Situations**:

- **Challenge**: Navigating social events, dining out, and holidays while sticking to your carb cycling plan.

- **Solution**: Plan ahead by reviewing menus, bringing your own healthy dishes to gatherings, and allowing for occasional flexibility. Communicate your goals with friends and family for support.

3. **Cravings and Temptations**:

- **Challenge**: Managing cravings for high-carb or unhealthy foods on low carb days.

- **Solution**: Keep healthy, low-carb snacks on hand, stay hydrated, and find alternative activities to distract from cravings. Allow for occasional treats in moderation to avoid feeling deprived.

4. **Plateaus and Lack of Progress**:

- **Challenge**: Hitting a plateau or not seeing expected results.
- **Solution**: Reevaluate your plan, adjust carb cycling frequency, macronutrient ratios, and caloric intake, and vary your workouts. Consider seeking professional guidance if needed.

5. **Fatigue and Energy Levels**:

- **Challenge**: Feeling fatigued or lacking energy on low carb days.
- **Solution**: Ensure you're consuming adequate protein and healthy fats, stay hydrated, and prioritize sleep. Consider timing your low carb days around less intense activities or rest days.

## Staying Motivated

Maintaining motivation is key to long-term success with carb cycling. Here are some strategies to help you stay motivated and committed:

1. **Set Clear Goals**:

   - Define specific, measurable, achievable, relevant, and time-bound (SMART) goals to give yourself clear direction and purpose.
   - Break larger goals into smaller milestones to celebrate progress along the way.

2. **Track Your Progress**:

   - Use a journal, app, or tracking sheet to log your workouts, meals, and progress metrics.
   - Regularly review your progress to stay accountable and motivated by seeing how far you've come.

3. **Find Support**:

   - Connect with a supportive community, whether online or in person, to share experiences, tips, and encouragement.

- Consider partnering with a friend or family member who shares similar goals for mutual support and accountability.

4. **Reward Yourself**:

- Set up a reward system to celebrate your achievements, such as treating yourself to a massage, new workout gear, or a fun activity.

- Use non-food rewards to reinforce positive behavior and maintain motivation.

5. **Stay Flexible**:

- Allow for flexibility in your plan to accommodate life's ups and downs. Remember that occasional deviations won't derail your progress as long as you stay consistent overall.

- Be kind to yourself and practice self-compassion when facing setbacks.

6. **Visualize Success**:

- Use visualization techniques to imagine yourself achieving your goals and enjoying the benefits of your hard work.
- Create a vision board with images and affirmations that inspire and motivate you.

## Building Long-Term Habits

Successful carb cycling involves building sustainable habits that support your long-term health and fitness goals. Here are some tips for creating lasting habits:

1. **Start Small**:

- Begin with small, manageable changes that you can gradually build upon over time. This makes it easier to stay consistent and avoid feeling overwhelmed.

2. **Create Routines**:

- Establish daily and weekly routines that incorporate your carb cycling plan, such as meal prep days, workout schedules, and regular progress check-ins.

- Consistent routines help reinforce positive habits and make them second nature.

3. **Focus on Enjoyment**:

- Choose foods and activities that you enjoy to make the process more enjoyable and sustainable.

- Experiment with new recipes, workouts, and hobbies to keep things interesting and prevent boredom.

4. **Reflect and Adjust**:

- Regularly reflect on your habits, progress, and challenges to identify areas for improvement.

- Be open to making adjustments to your plan as needed to better align with your goals and lifestyle.

Overcoming challenges and staying motivated are essential for long-term success with carb cycling. By implementing practical strategies for managing common obstacles, staying motivated, and building sustainable habits, you can achieve your health and fitness goals and maintain them for the long term.

# Chapter 8: Case Studies and Success Stories

Real-life examples of individuals who have successfully implemented carb cycling can provide valuable insights and inspiration. This chapter will share a range of case studies and success stories, highlighting different goals, strategies, and outcomes. These examples will demonstrate the versatility and effectiveness of carb cycling for various individuals.

## Case Study 1: John's Weight Loss Journey

**Background**: John, a 35-year-old office worker, struggled with obesity and related health issues, including high blood pressure and pre-diabetes. Weighing 250 pounds at 5'9", John decided to make a significant lifestyle change to improve his health and reduce his weight.

**Goals**:

- Lose 60 pounds over one year.

- Improve blood pressure and blood sugar levels.
- Increase energy levels and overall fitness.

**Plan**: John followed a carb cycling plan tailored for weight loss, combined with regular exercise:

- **High Carb Days**: 2 days per week (Monday, Thursday) with intense strength training.
- **Low Carb Days**: 3 days per week (Tuesday, Wednesday, Friday) with light cardio or rest.
- **Moderate Carb Days**: 2 days per week (Saturday, Sunday) with moderate activity, such as hiking or swimming.

**Results**:

- **Weight Loss**: John lost 65 pounds in 12 months, exceeding his goal.
- **Health Improvements**: His blood pressure and blood sugar levels normalized.

- **Fitness Gains**: John's energy levels increased, and he gained muscle mass.

**Key Takeaways**:

- Consistency with meal prep and exercise was crucial.

- Regular monitoring and adjustments helped overcome plateaus.

- Support from family and friends provided motivation and accountability.

## Case Study 2: Sarah's Muscle Gain and Performance Enhancement

**Background**: Sarah, a 28-year-old competitive athlete, aimed to improve her performance and increase lean muscle mass. She was already in good shape but wanted to optimize her diet to support her training and competition schedule.

**Goals**:

- Gain 10 pounds of lean muscle mass over six months.

- Enhance athletic performance in track and field events.
- Improve recovery and reduce muscle soreness.

**Plan**: Sarah implemented a carb cycling plan focused on muscle gain and performance:

- **High Carb Days**: 3 days per week (Monday, Wednesday, Saturday) with intense training sessions, including weightlifting and sprinting.
- **Low Carb Days**: 2 days per week (Tuesday, Thursday) with light recovery workouts, such as yoga and stretching.
- **Moderate Carb Days**: 2 days per week (Friday, Sunday) with moderate training, like steady-state cardio and technique drills.

**Results**:

- **Muscle Gain**: Sarah gained 12 pounds of lean muscle mass in six months.

- **Performance Enhancement**: She set personal records in her events and improved her competitive rankings.
- **Recovery**: Reduced muscle soreness and faster recovery times between workouts.

**Key Takeaways**:

- Strategic carb intake around training sessions boosted performance and recovery.

- A balanced approach to macronutrients ensured muscle growth and overall health.

- Flexibility in the plan allowed Sarah to adjust for competition schedules and rest periods.

## Case Study 3: Emily's Improved Energy and Hormonal Balance

**Background**: Emily, a 42-year-old mother of two, experienced chronic fatigue and hormonal imbalances, including thyroid issues and irregular menstrual cycles. She sought a dietary approach to help regulate her hormones and increase her energy levels.

## Goals:

- Regulate hormonal balance and improve menstrual cycle regularity.
- Increase daily energy levels and reduce fatigue.
- Enhance overall well-being and mental clarity.

**Plan**: Emily followed a carb cycling plan designed for hormonal balance and energy:

- **High Carb Days**: 1 day per week (Saturday) focused on rest and family activities.
- **Low Carb Days**: 4 days per week (Monday, Wednesday, Friday, Sunday) with gentle activities, like walking and Pilates.
- **Moderate Carb Days**: 2 days per week (Tuesday, Thursday) with moderate exercise, such as biking or swimming.

**Results**:

- **Hormonal Balance**: Improved thyroid function and regular menstrual cycles within three months.
- **Increased Energy**: Significant reduction in fatigue and improved daily energy levels.
- **Enhanced Well-Being**: Better mental clarity, mood, and overall well-being.

**Key Takeaways**:

- Emphasizing nutrient-dense foods and balanced macronutrient intake supported hormonal health.

- Listening to her body and adjusting carb intake based on energy needs helped manage fatigue.

- Combining carb cycling with stress-reduction techniques, like mindfulness and adequate sleep, contributed to overall improvements.

## Case Study 4: Mike's Body Recomposition

**Background**: Mike, a 30-year-old fitness enthusiast, wanted to achieve body recomposition by losing fat while gaining muscle. Despite regular workouts, he struggled to see significant changes in his body composition.

**Goals**:

- Reduce body fat percentage from 20% to 12% over eight months.
- Gain 5-10 pounds of lean muscle mass.
- Improve muscle definition and overall physique.

**Plan**: Mike adopted a carb cycling plan focused on body recomposition:

- **High Carb Days**: 2 days per week (Wednesday, Saturday) with heavy strength training and high-intensity workouts.
- **Low Carb Days**: 3 days per week (Monday, Thursday, Sunday) with low-intensity cardio and active recovery.

- **Moderate Carb Days**: 2 days per week (Tuesday, Friday) with moderate strength training and conditioning.

**Results**:

- **Body Fat Reduction**: Decreased body fat percentage to 11% in eight months.
- **Muscle Gain**: Gained 8 pounds of lean muscle mass.
- **Improved Physique**: Achieved greater muscle definition and a more athletic build.

**Key Takeaways**:

- Tailoring carb intake to workout intensity supported fat loss and muscle gain.

- Regular progress tracking and photo comparisons provided motivation and insight.

- Incorporating a variety of exercises prevented plateaus and promoted balanced development.

These case studies demonstrate the diverse applications and benefits of carb cycling for weight loss, muscle gain, performance enhancement, hormonal balance, and body recomposition. By tailoring carb cycling plans to individual goals and needs, anyone can achieve significant improvements in their health and fitness.

# Chapter 9: Carb Cycling for Different Populations

Carb cycling can be adapted for various populations with unique needs, such as athletes, vegetarians, older adults, and individuals with specific health conditions. This chapter will explore how to tailor carb cycling for different groups to maximize benefits and ensure safety.

## Athletes and Active Individuals

Athletes and highly active individuals often require higher carbohydrate intake to support their energy needs, performance, and recovery.

**Strategies**:

1. **Increased High Carb Days**:

   - Schedule high carb days around intense training sessions and competitions to optimize glycogen stores and performance.

- Ensure sufficient carbohydrate intake during and after workouts to support recovery.

## 2. Balanced Macronutrient Ratios:

- Maintain a balanced intake of protein and fats to support muscle repair, hormone production, and overall health.
- Monitor individual responses to carb cycling and adjust as needed to prevent fatigue and overtraining.

## Example Plan:

- **High Carb Days**: 3-4 days per week with intense training.
- **Moderate Carb Days**: 2-3 days per week with moderate training or rest.
- **Low Carb Days**: 1 day per week for active recovery or rest.

## Vegetarians and Vegans

Vegetarians and vegans can successfully implement carb cycling by focusing on plant-based sources of carbohydrates, protein, and fats.

**Strategies**:

1. **High-Quality Plant Proteins**:

   - Incorporate a variety of plant-based protein sources, such as legumes, tofu, tempeh, seitan, and protein-rich grains.
   - Use protein powders, such as pea or hemp protein, to meet daily protein needs.

2. **Complex Carbohydrates**:

   - Emphasize whole grains, fruits, vegetables, and legumes for carbohydrate intake.
   - Avoid highly processed carbs and focus on nutrient-dense options.

**Example Plan**:

- **High Carb Days**: 2-3 days per week with plant-based protein sources and complex carbs.

- **Moderate Carb Days**: 2-3 days per week with balanced intake of protein, carbs, and fats.
- **Low Carb Days**: 2-3 days per week with higher emphasis on non-starchy vegetables and plant-based fats.

## Older Adults

Older adults may benefit from carb cycling to support healthy aging, maintain muscle mass, and manage weight and metabolic health.

**Strategies**:

1. **Protein Prioritization**:

   - Ensure adequate protein intake to support muscle maintenance and repair.
   - Include high-quality protein sources at each meal, such as lean meats, fish, eggs, dairy, and plant-based options.

2. **Moderate Carb Intake**:

- Focus on moderate carb intake to support energy levels and cognitive function.
- Emphasize nutrient-dense carbohydrates, such as fruits, vegetables, and whole grains.

**Example Plan**:

- **High Carb Days**: 1-2 days per week with gentle strength training or physical activity.
- **Moderate Carb Days**: 3-4 days per week with moderate activity, such as walking or swimming.
- **Low Carb Days**: 1-2 days per week with focus on healthy fats and non-starchy vegetables.

## Individuals with Specific Health Conditions

Carb cycling can be adapted to support individuals with conditions such as diabetes, metabolic syndrome, or thyroid issues. Always consult with a healthcare provider before making dietary changes.

**Strategies**:

1. **Diabetes and Metabolic Syndrome**:

   - Emphasize low and moderate carb days to manage blood sugar levels.
   - Include high-fiber foods and avoid refined sugars and processed carbs.

2. **Thyroid Issues**:

   - Ensure balanced intake of macronutrients to support thyroid function.
   - Avoid extreme low carb days and maintain moderate carb intake to prevent metabolic stress.

**Example Plan for Diabetes**:

- **High Carb Days**: 1 day per week with balanced meals and complex carbs.

- **Moderate Carb Days**: 3-4 days per week with moderate carb intake and focus on fiber.
- **Low Carb Days**: 2-3 days per week with emphasis on healthy fats and protein.

**Example Plan for Thyroid Issues**:

- **High Carb Days**: 1-2 days per week with nutrient-dense carbs and balanced meals.
- **Moderate Carb Days**: 3-4 days per week with focus on overall nutrient intake.
- **Low Carb Days**: 1-2 days per week with moderate carb intake and healthy fats.

Carb cycling can be tailored to meet the unique needs of various populations, providing flexibility and effectiveness for diverse dietary requirements and health goals. By understanding and applying specific strategies, individuals can optimize their carb cycling plans to support their overall well-being.

# Chapter 10: Frequently Asked Questions (FAQs)

This chapter addresses common questions about carb cycling, providing clear and concise answers to help you better understand and implement this dietary approach.

## What is carb cycling?

Carb cycling is a dietary approach that alternates between high, moderate, and low carbohydrate intake on different days to optimize metabolic function, support physical activity, and achieve specific health and fitness goals.

## How does carb cycling work?

Carb cycling works by manipulating carbohydrate intake to match energy needs and metabolic processes. High carb days provide glycogen replenishment and energy for intense workouts, while low carb days promote fat burning and insulin sensitivity.

## Who can benefit from carb cycling?

Carb cycling can benefit various individuals, including those looking to lose weight, gain muscle, enhance athletic performance, improve metabolic health, and manage specific health conditions. It is adaptable to different lifestyles and dietary preferences.

## Is carb cycling safe?

Carb cycling is generally safe for most healthy individuals. However, it's important to consult with a healthcare provider before starting, especially if you have any medical conditions or concerns. Pregnant or breastfeeding women should seek medical advice before making significant dietary changes.

## How do I start carb cycling?

To start carb cycling:

1. Determine your goals (e.g., weight loss, muscle gain, performance).

2. Plan your carb cycling schedule (e.g., high, moderate, low carb days).

3. Calculate your macronutrient needs for each type of day.

4. Plan and prepare meals according to your schedule and macronutrient targets.

5. Monitor your progress and adjust as needed.

## What foods should I eat on high carb days?

On high carb days, focus on nutrient-dense, complex carbohydrates, such as:

- Whole grains (e.g., oats, quinoa, brown rice)
- Fruits (e.g., berries, apples, bananas)
- Starchy vegetables (e.g., sweet potatoes, squash, corn)
- Legumes (e.g., beans, lentils)
- Lean proteins and healthy fats to balance meals.

## What foods should I eat on low carb days?

On low carb days, prioritize:

- Non-starchy vegetables (e.g., leafy greens, broccoli, peppers)
- Lean proteins (e.g., chicken, fish, tofu)
- Healthy fats (e.g., avocados, nuts, seeds, olive oil)
- Limited amounts of low-sugar fruits (e.g., berries).

## How do I adjust carb cycling for different fitness goals?

Adjust carb cycling based on your fitness goals:

- **Weight Loss**: More low carb days to promote fat burning.
- **Muscle Gain**: More high carb days to support muscle growth and recovery.

- **Performance Enhancement**: Balanced approach with high carb days around intense training sessions.

## Can I do carb cycling if I'm vegetarian or vegan?

Yes, vegetarians and vegans can successfully implement carb cycling by focusing on plant-based sources of carbohydrates, proteins, and fats. Use a variety of plant-based foods to meet nutritional needs and ensure adequate protein intake.

## How do I handle social situations and dining out?

Plan ahead by reviewing menus, choosing restaurants with healthy options, and communicating your dietary preferences with friends and family. Allow for occasional flexibility and balance to enjoy social events without feeling restricted.

## How do I track progress with carb cycling?

Track progress using:

- Body weight and measurements
- Progress photos
- Performance metrics (e.g., workout logs)
- Food diaries or nutrition tracking apps
- Health markers (e.g., blood sugar, cholesterol)

**What should I do if I hit a plateau?**

If you hit a plateau, consider:

- Adjusting carb cycling frequency and macronutrient ratios.
- Modifying workout intensity and variety.
- Ensuring adequate rest and recovery.
- Seeking professional guidance if needed.

**Can carb cycling help with hormonal balance?**

Yes, carb cycling can support hormonal balance by providing adequate nutrients and energy, reducing metabolic stress, and improving insulin sensitivity. It can be particularly beneficial for managing conditions like thyroid issues and PCOS.

## How long should I follow a carb cycling plan?

The duration of carb cycling depends on your goals and individual response. Some people use it as a short-term strategy to achieve specific goals, while others incorporate it as a long-term lifestyle approach. Regularly evaluate your progress and adjust as needed.

## Is carb cycling suitable for everyone?

Carb cycling may not be suitable for everyone, particularly those with certain medical conditions, eating disorders, or specific dietary restrictions. Always consult with a healthcare provider before starting a new dietary approach to ensure it aligns with your health needs.

Carb cycling is a flexible and effective dietary strategy that can be tailored to various goals, lifestyles, and health needs. By addressing common questions and providing practical answers, this chapter aims to equip you with the knowledge and confidence to successfully implement carb cycling in your life.

# Chapter 11: Conclusion and Next Steps

Carb cycling offers a versatile and effective approach to achieving a variety of health and fitness goals. This chapter will summarize the key points covered in the book and provide guidance on taking the next steps to implement and sustain a successful carb cycling plan.

## Summary of Key Points

1. **Understanding Carb Cycling**:

   - Carb cycling alternates between high, moderate, and low carbohydrate intake to optimize metabolic function, support physical activity, and achieve specific goals.

2. **Benefits of Carb Cycling**:

   - Supports weight loss, muscle gain, performance enhancement, hormonal balance, and overall health.

- Adaptable to different populations, including athletes, vegetarians, older adults, and those with specific health conditions.

3. **Implementing Carb Cycling**:

   - Determine your goals and create a tailored carb cycling schedule.
   - Calculate macronutrient needs and plan meals accordingly.
   - Incorporate regular exercise, focusing on different workout intensities to match carb intake.

4. **Monitoring Progress and Adjustments**:

   - Track key metrics, such as body weight, measurements, performance, and health markers.
   - Regularly evaluate the effectiveness of your plan and make informed adjustments.

5. **Overcoming Challenges and Staying Motivated**:

- Address common challenges with practical strategies.

- Maintain motivation through goal setting, tracking progress, finding support, and building sustainable habits.

6. **Tailoring Carb Cycling for Different Populations**:

- Adapt carb cycling plans to meet the unique needs of athletes, vegetarians, older adults, and individuals with specific health conditions.

7. **Frequently Asked Questions**:

- Provide clear answers to common questions about carb cycling, helping you better understand and implement this dietary approach.

## Next Steps

1. **Set Clear Goals**:

   - Define your health and fitness goals, ensuring they are specific, measurable, achievable, relevant, and time-bound (SMART).

2. **Create Your Plan**:

   - Develop a carb cycling schedule that aligns with your goals and lifestyle.
   - Calculate your macronutrient needs for high, moderate, and low carb days.

3. **Plan and Prepare Meals**:

   - Plan and prepare meals in advance to ensure adherence to your carb cycling plan.
   - Use recipes and meal ideas provided in this book to keep your diet enjoyable and varied.

4. **Incorporate Regular Exercise**:

- Design a workout program that complements your carb cycling schedule.
- Include a mix of high-intensity, moderate-intensity, and low-intensity activities.

5. **Monitor Your Progress**:

- Regularly track your progress using body measurements, photos, performance metrics, and health markers.
- Adjust your plan as needed based on your progress and feedback from your body.

6. **Stay Motivated**:

- Set up a support system, find a fitness buddy, or join a community to stay motivated.
- Celebrate your achievements and maintain a positive mindset.

7. **Seek Professional Guidance**:

- Consider consulting with a nutritionist, dietitian, or fitness coach for personalized advice and support.

- Regular check-ups with your healthcare provider can help monitor health markers and ensure your plan is safe and effective.

## Final Thoughts

Carb cycling is a powerful tool that can help you achieve your health and fitness goals, whether you're looking to lose weight, gain muscle, enhance performance, or improve overall well-being. By understanding the principles of carb cycling, implementing a tailored plan, and staying committed to your goals, you can experience significant and lasting results.

Remember the Do The Easy Fitness motto – "Choosing What Motivate You Makes Things Easier". Be patient, stay consistent, stay motivated and enjoy the process of discovering what works best for you. If need be, then mix things up until you find the right combination that works for you. With the knowledge and strategies provided in this book, you are well equipped to embark on a successful carb cycling journey and transform your health and fitness.

Good luck, from Do The Easy Fitness and Thank You for Your Support!